SO-CNI-270

QUICK REFERENCE TO COMMUNITY HEALTH NURSING

MARCIA STANHOPE, RN, DSN, FAAN

Professor and Director
Division of Community Health Nursing
   and Administration
College of Nursing, University of Kentucky
Lexington, Kentucky

JEANETTE LANCASTER, RN, PhD, FAAN

Dean and Sadie Heath Cabaniss Professor
School of Nursing, University of Virginia
Charlottesville, Virginia

Acknowledgments to
Ruth Knollmueller, RN, PhD

Second Edition

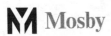 Mosby

St. Louis   Baltimore   Boston
Carlsbad   Chicago   Naples   New York   Philadelphia   Portland
London   Madrid   Mexico City   Singapore   Sydney   Tokyo   Toronto   Wiesbaden

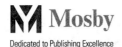
Mosby

Dedicated to Publishing Excellence

Publisher: Nancy L. Coon
Editor: Loren Wilson
Associate Developmental Editor: Brian Dennison
Project Manager: Patricia Tannian
Senior Production Editor: Betty Hazelwood
Book Design Manager: Gail Morey Hudson
Manufacturing Manager: David Graybill

SECOND EDITION

Copyright © 1996 by Mosby–Year Book, Inc.

Previous edition copyrighted 1993

Printed in the United States of America
Composition by Top Graphics
Printing/binding by Plus Communications

Mosby–Year Book, Inc.
11830 Westline Industrial Drive
St. Louis, Missouri 63146

International Standard Book Number 0-8151-8335-6

99 / 9 8 7 6 5 4 3

CONTENTS

ENVIRONMENTAL ASSESSMENT
HOME ASSESSMENT CHECKLIST
General Household

1. Is there good lighting available, especially around stairwells?
2. Are there handrails (that can be easily grasped) on both sides of the staircases, designed to indicate when top and bottom steps have been reached?
3. Are top and bottom steps painted in easily seen colors? Are nonskid treads used?
4. Are the edges of rugs tacked down? (Suggest the use of wall-to-wall carpeting.)
5. Is a telephone present? Does the telephone have a dial that is easily readable? Are emergency numbers written in large print and kept near the telephone?
6. Are electrical cords, footstools, and other low-lying objects kept out of walkways?
7. Are electrical cords in good condition?
8. Is furniture arranged to allow for free movement in heavily traveled areas?
9. Is furniture sturdy enough to give support?

From Tideiksaar R: Ritter Department of Geriatrics and Adult Development, The Mount Sinai Medical Center, New York, 1993.

10. Is furniture designed to accommodate easy transfers on and off?
11. Is the temperature of the home within a comfortable range?
12. If fireplaces or other heating devices are present, do they have protective screens?
13. Are smoke detectors present (especially in the kitchen and bedroom)?
14. Are rapidly closing doors eliminated?
15. Are there alternative exits from the house?
16. Are basements and attics easy to get to, well lighted, and well ventilated?
17. Are slippers and shoes in good repair? Do they fit properly and have nonskid soles?

Kitchen
18. Are there loose extension cords, small sliding rugs, slippery linoleum tiles present? (Suggest the use of rubber-backed, nonskid rugs and nonskid floor wax.)
19. Is the cooking stove gas or electric?
20. Are there large easily readable dials present on the stove or other appliances, with the "on" and "off" positions clearly marked?
21. Are refrigerators in good working order? Are refrigerators placed on 18-inch platforms to avoid bending over?
22. Are spaces for food storage adequate? Are shelves at eye level and easily reachable?
23. Is a sturdy stepladder present for reaching?
24. Are electrical circuits overloaded with too many appliances?
25. Are electrical appliances disconnected when not in use?
26. Are sharp objects (such as carving knives) kept in special holders?
27. Are cleaning fluids, polishes, bleaches, detergents, and all poisons stored separately and clearly marked?

28. Are kitchen chairs sturdy, with arm rests and high backs?
29. Is stove free from flammable objects?
30. Are pot holders available for removing pots and pans from the stove?
31. Is baking soda available in case of fire?

Bathroom
32. Are there grab bars in the bath, in the shower, and around the toilet?
33. Are toilet seats high enough to get on and off without difficulty?
34. Can the bathroom door be easily closed to ensure privacy? (Avoid locks.)
35. Are bathroom doorways wide enough for easy wheelchair and walker access?
36. Are there nonskid rubber mats in the bath, in the shower, and on the floor?
37. Is there good lighting in the area of the medicine cabinet?
38. Are internal and external medications stored separately? And safely (especially important with young grandchildren present in the house)?
39. Do medication containers have childproof tops? Are they labeled in large print? Is a magnifying glass present for reading medication instructions?
40. Have all outdated medications been discarded?
41. Do you notice any medications (both prescription and over-the-counter) that could cause adverse side effects or drug-drug interactions that the patient is unaware of?
42. Can the water temperature be easily regulated?
43. Are electrical cords, outlets, and appliances a safe distance from the tub?

44. Are razor blades kept in a safe place?
45. Is a first aid kit available?

Bedroom

46. Is there adequate lighting from the bedside to the bathroom?
47. Are lights easily accessible? (If not, suggest keeping a flashlight by the bedside or using a flashlight for entry into dark rooms if light switch is not within easy reach.)
48. Are beds in good repair?
49. Are beds at the proper height to allow for easy transfer on and off without difficulty?
50. Do bedroom rugs have nonskid rubber backings?

CULTURAL ASSESSMENT
SOCIOCULTURAL FACTORS IN COMMUNITY ASSESSMENT

1. Existing influences that divide people into groups within the community, such as ethnicity, religion, social class, occupation, place of residence, language, education, sex, race, and age
2. Conditions that lead to social conflict and/or social cohesion
3. Attitudes toward minority groups, youth and the elderly, males and females, and age and gender groups
4. Division of the community into neighborhoods or districts and the characteristics of these
5. Formal and informal channels of communication between health programs and the community
6. Barriers that may be the result of differences in cultural beliefs and practices
7. Political orientation in the community (attitudes toward authority and its use in health problems)
8. Patterns of migration either in or out of a community and their effect on health care services
9. Relation of religion and medicine within the community (who and what causes various illnesses and how they can be prevented)
10. Types of diseases or illnesses thought by various members of the community to exist (culture-specific conditions, such as illnesses caused by hot and cold imbalances or diseases of magical origin)

Developed by E Bawens and S Anderson from Brownlee AT: *Community, culture, and care,* St Louis, 1978, Mosby.

FAMILY ASSESSMENT
FAMILY COPING INDEX
Scaling Cues

The following descriptive statements are "cues" to help you as you rate family coping. They are limited to three points: *1,* or no competence; *3,* moderate competence; and *5,* complete competence. You will find, however, that most families will fall somewhere in between these points. Mark the point you feel most nearly describes the level of competence they have. The descriptions are not complete but suggestive. In the long run it is your own professional judgment that will be needed to make a decision. When there is no problem or the area is not relevant, check the "no problem" column.

1. Physical Independence

This category is concerned with ability to move about, to get in and out of bed, to take care of daily grooming, walking, etc. Note that it is the *family* competence that is measured—even though an individual is dependent, if the family is able to compensate for this the family may be independent. However, the quality, as well as quantity, of ability is important; hence, if the *focus* of care is poor—if a mother is giving care to a handicapped child that the child could give himself, or if one person is given care that should be shared with other members—the independence might be considered incomplete. The *causes* of dependence may vary—lack of physical independence in the family may be due to actual physical incapacity, to lack of "know-how," to unwillingness or fear of doing the necessary tasks.

Developed jointly by the Richmond IVNA City Nursing Service and the Johns Hopkins School of Hygiene and Public Health, 1964.

1 = Family failing entirely to provide required personal care to one or more of its members. *Example:* arthritic client unable to get out of bed alone, no one available to help; client "cannot" give his hypodermic medication because of fear.

3 = Family providing partially for needs of its members, or providing care for some members but not for others. *Example:* mother may be doing well with own and husband's care, but failing to give daily care efficiently to newborn baby; daughter may be giving excellent physical care to aged mother but at cost of neglecting children somewhat, or with poor body mechanics that place undue strain upon herself.

5 = All family members, whether or not there is infirmity or disability in one or more members, are receiving the necessary care to maintain cleanliness, including skin care, are able to get about as far as possible within their physical abilities; are receiving assistance when needed without interruption or undue delay.

2. Therapeutic Competence

This category includes all of the procedures or treatment prescribed for the care of illness such as giving medications, using appliances (including crutches), dressings, exercises and relaxation, special diets, etc.

1 = Family either not carrying out procedures prescribed or doing it unsafely. For example, giving several medications without being able to distinguish one from the other, or taking them inappropriately; applying braces so they throw the limb out of line; measuring insulin incorrectly. Family resents, rejects, or refuses to give necessary care.

3 = Family carrying out some but not all of the treatments—for example, giving insulin but not adhering strictly to diet; carrying

out procedures awkwardly, ineffectively, or with resentment or unnecessary anxiety. For example, crutch walking may be done, but with the helper using poor body mechanics, or not giving the client enough security and confidence; client may give own hypodermic, but say "I dread it every time." May be giving medications correctly, but not understanding purposes of the drug or symptoms to be observed.

5 = Family able to demonstrate that they can carry out the prescribed procedures safely and efficiently, with the understanding of the principles involved and with a confident and willing attitude.

3. Knowledge of Health Condition

This category is concerned with the particular health condition that is the occasion for care. For example, knowledge of the disease or disability, understanding of communicability of disease and modes of transmission, understanding of general pattern of development of a newborn baby and the basic needs of infants for physical care and TLC.

1 = Totally uninformed or misinformed about the condition. For example, believes tuberculosis is caused by sin, or syphilis cured when symptoms subside; believes stroke patient must be bedridden, and that it is cruel to make them do for themselves; that overweight in the school-age child is "healthy."

3 = Has some general knowledge of the disease or condition, but has not grasped the underlying principles, or is only partially informed. For instance, may recognize need for TLC but not relate this to placing the baby's crib near people when the baby is awake or holding the baby when feeding; may accept fact that client is dying but not see need to prepare family for this event;

may understand dietary and insulin control of diabetes, but not need for special care of feet, etc.

5 = Knows the salient facts about the disease well enough to take necessary action at the proper time, understands the rationale of care, able to observe and report significant symptoms.

4. Application of Principles of Personal and General Hygiene

This is concerned with family action in relation to maintaining family nutrition, securing adequate rest and relaxation for family members, carrying out accepted preventive measures such as immunizations, medical appraisal, and safe homemaking habits in relation to storing and preparing food.

1 = Family diet grossly inadequate or unbalanced, necessary immunizations not secured for children; house dirty, food handled in unsanitary way; members of family working beyond reasonable limits; children and adults getting too little sleep; family members unkempt, dirty, inadequately clothed in relation to weather.

3 = Failing to apply some general principles of hygiene—for instance, keeping house in excellent condition but expending too much energy and becoming overfatigued as a result; secured initial immunizations but not boosters, or some but not all available immunizations; general diet and homemaking skills good, but father carrying two full-time jobs.

5 = Household runs smoothly, family meals well selected; habits of sleep and rest adequate to needs.

5. Health Care Attitudes

This category is concerned with the way the family feels about health care in general, including preventive services, care of illness, and public health measures.

1 = Family resents and resists all health care; has no confidence in physicians, uses patent medicines and quack nostrums, feels illness is unavoidable and to be borne rather than treated; feels community health agencies shouldn't interfere or bother them; practices folk medicine or superstitious rites in illness.

3 = Accepts health care in some degree, but with reservations. For example, may accept need for medical care for illness, but not general preventive measures; may have confidence in physicians generally, but not in the clinic or "free" physicians; may feel certain illnesses are hopeless (such as cancer), or care unnecessary—for instance, dental care for the young child.

5 = Understands and recognizes need for medical care in illness and for the usual preventive services, arranges for periodic physical appraisals and follows through with recommendations, accepts illness calmly and recognizes the limits it imposes while doing all possible to effect recovery and rehabilitation.

6. Emotional Competence

This category has to do with the maturity and integrity with which the members of the family are able to meet the usual stresses and problems of life, and to plan for happy and fruitful living. The degree to which individuals accept the necessary disciplines imposed by one's family and culture; the development and maintenance of individual responsibility and decision; willingness to meet reasonable obligations, to accept diversity with fortitude, to consider the needs of others as well as one's own.

1 = Family does not face realities—assumes moribund client will get well, that they can eventually pay a hospital bill far beyond their means, that an unwanted pregnancy isn't so; one or more members lacking in any emotional control—uncontrollable rages, irresponsible sexual activities; one or more members alcoholic, family torn, suspicious of one another; evidences of great insecurity, guilt, or anxiety.

3 = Family members usually do fairly well, but one or more members evidence lack of security or maturity. For example, thumb sucking in late childhood; unusual concern with what the neighbors will think; failure to plan ahead for foreseeable emergencies; leaving children unattended, "fighting" in the family on occasion.

5 = All members of the family are able to maintain a reasonable degree of emotional calm, face up to illness realistically and hopefully; able to discuss problems and differences with objectivity and reasonable emotional control; do not worry unduly about trivial matters, consider the needs and wishes of other family members, of neighbors and those with whom they work and live in making decisions or deciding upon action.

7. Family Living Patterns

This category is concerned largely with the interpersonal or group aspects of family life—how well the members of the family get along with one another, the ways in which they make decisions affecting the family as a whole, the degree to which they support one another and do things as a family, the degree of respect and affection they show for one another, the ways in which they manage the family budget, the kind of discipline that prevails.

1 = Family consists of a group of individuals indifferent or hostile to one another, or strongly dominated and controlled by a single family member; no control of children, or family so totally dependent on one another that they are being stifled—for example, mother developing habits of dependence in sons so as to threaten future capacity for independence in own family life, no rational plan for managing available money; "battered" child.

3 = Family gets along but has habits or customs that interfere with their effectiveness or coherence as a family. For example, a family fond of one another, have many home activities, but dominated by a father in a kindly way; recreational habits separate family much of the time; children somewhat overprotected; expectations of the children unrealistic—parents expecting children with low academic competence to enter professions, etc.

5 = Family cohesive, does things together, each member acts with regard for the good of the family as a whole; children respect parents and vice versa; family tasks shared; evidence of planning.

8. Physical Environment

This category is concerned with the home and community or work environment as it affects family health. The condition for housing, presence of accident hazards, screening, plumbing, facilities for cooking and for privacy; level of community—(deteriorated or modern, presence of social hazards such as bars, street gangs, delinquency, pests such as rats), availability and condition of schools, transportation.

1 = House in poor condition, unsafe, unscreened, poorly heated, neighborhood deteriorated, juvenile and adult delinquency among neighbors, no play space except streets.

3 = House needs some repair or painting but fundamentally sound; neighborhood poor but possible to protect children from social influence through school or other community activities; house crowded but adjustments to this fairly adequate.

5 = House in good repair, provides for privacy for members and is free of accidents and pest hazards; neighborhood respectable and provided with play space for children; free from undesirable social elements; opportunities for community activity.

9. Use of Community Facilities

This category has to do with the degree to which the family knows about and the wisdom with which they use available community resources for health, education, and welfare. This would include the ways in which they use services of private physicians, clinics, emergency rooms, hospitals, schools, welfare organizations, churches, and so forth. The *coping ability* does not indicate the level of the *need* for services, but rather the degree to which they can cope when they must seek such aid. Even though a family has a severe housing problem, if they have used all appropriate facilities for enforcing landlord's compliance with sanitary regulations to secure public housing, their coping capacity in relation to *use* of community facilities is high, even though the underlying condition is not corrected.

1 = Family has obvious and serious social needs, but has not sought or found any help for them. For example, a family may be borrowing unreasonable sums of money for medical care, while not using available free hospitals or clinics; or leaving children without any supervision while the mother works; or fail to take steps to register for public housing when it is indicated. Using resources inappropriately, for example, calling ambulance or using emergency services for minor ills.

3 = Family knows about or uses some, but not all of the available community resources that they need. For example, the family may be under welfare care, and know how to use the social worker responsible for their care, but not have recognized that

the counselor in the school could help with educational planning, or that the church might provide recreational activities for the children as well as spiritual guidance.

5 = Family using the facilities they need appropriately and promptly. Know when to call for help and whom to call. Feel secure in their relationship with community workers such as social workers, teachers, physicians, etc.

Family Coping Estimate

Family _____ Nurse _____ Date _____

Initial _____ Periodic _____ Discharge _____

Coping area	Rating x-status 0-est. change Poor .... Exc.	Justification
Physical independence	1 2 3 4 5 Not applicable ☐	
Therapeutic independence	1 2 3 4 5 Not applicable ☐	
Knowledge of condition	1 2 3 4 5 Not applicable ☐	
Application of principles of hygiene	1 2 3 4 5 Not applicable ☐	
Attitude toward health care	1 2 3 4 5 Not applicable ☐	
Emotional competence	1 2 3 4 5 Not applicable ☐	
Family living patterns	1 2 3 4 5 Not applicable ☐	
Physical environment	1 2 3 4 5 Not applicable ☐	
Use of community resources	1 2 3 4 5 Not applicable ☐	

Comments

CHILD ASSESSMENT
PEDIATRIC HEALTH HISTORY
Identifying Information
1. Name
2. Address
3. Telephone number
4. Age and birthdate
5. Birthplace
6. Race
7. Sex
8. Religion
9. Nationality
10. Date of interview
11. Informant

Additional information appropriate to older adolescent may include occupation, marital status, and temporary and permanent address.

Under informant include subjective impression of reliability, general attitude, willingness to communicate, overall accuracy of data, and any special circumstances, such as use of an interpreter.

Informants should include parent and child, as well as others who may be primary caregivers, such as grandparent.

Chief Complaint (CC)
To establish the major specific reason for the individual's seeking professional health attention.

Record in client's own words; include duration of symptoms.

Modified from Wong DL, Whaley LF: *Essentials of pediatric nursing,* ed 4, St Louis, 1993, Mosby.

If informant has difficulty isolating *one* problem, ask which problem or symptom led person to seek help *now*.

In case of routine physical examination, state CC as reason for visit.

Present Illness (PI)

To obtain all details related to the chief complaint.

In its broadest sense, *illness* denotes any problem of a physical, emotional, or psychosocial nature.

1. Onset
   a. Date of onset
   b. Manner of onset (gradual or sudden)
   c. Precipitating and predisposing factors related to onset (emotional disturbance, physical exertion, fatigue, bodily function, pregnancy, environment, injury, infection, toxins and allergens, or therapeutic agents)
2. Characteristics
   a. Character (quality, quantity, consistency, or other)
   b. Location and radiation (i.e., pain)
   c. Intensity or severity
   d. Timing (continuous or intermittent, duration of each, temporal relationship to other events)
   e. Aggravating and relieving factors
   f. Associated symptoms

Present information in chronologic order; may be referenced according to one point in time, such as *prior to admission* (PTA).

3. Course since onset
   a. Incidence
      (1) Single acute attack
      (2) Recurrent acute attacks

      (3) Daily occurrences

      (4) Periodic occurrences

      (5) Continuous chronic episode

    b. Progress (better, worse, unchanged)

    c. Effect of therapy

Concentrate on reason for seeking help now, especially if problem has existed for some time.

Past History (PH)

    To elicit a profile of the individual's previous illnesses, injuries, or operations.

  1. Pregnancy (maternal)

    a. Number (gravida)

      (1) Dates of delivery

    b. Outcome (parity)

      (1) Gestation (full-term, premature, postmature)

      (2) Stillbirths, abortions

    c. Health during pregnancy

    d. Medications taken

Importance of perinatal history depends on child's age; the younger the child, the more important the perinatal history.

Explain relevance of obstetric history in revealing important factors relating to the child's health.

Assess parents' emotional attitudes toward the pregnancy and birth.

  2. Labor and delivery

    a. Duration of labor

    b. Type of delivery

    c. Place of delivery

    d. Medications

Assess parents' feelings regarding delivery; investigate factors affecting bonding, such as if awake and able to hold infant or if asleep and separated from infant.

3. Birth
   a. Weight and length
   b. Time of regaining birth weight
   c. Condition of health
   d. Apgar score
   e. Presence of congenital anomalies
   f. Date of discharge from nursery

If birth problems are reported, inquire about treatment, such as use of oxygen, phototherapy, surgery, and so on, and parents' emotional response to the event.

4. Previous illnesses, operations, or injuries
   a. Onset, symptoms, course, termination
   b. Occurrence of complications
   c. Incidence of disease in other family members or in community

Make positive statements about diphtheria, scarlet fever, measles, chickenpox, mumps, tonsillitis, pertussis, and common illnesses such as colds, earaches, or sore throats.

Elicit a description of disease to verify the diagnosis.

   d. Emotional response to previous hospitalization
   e. Circumstances and nature of injuries

Be alert to areas of injury prevention.

5. Allergies
   a. Hay fever, asthma, or eczema

Have parent describe the type of allergic reaction.

    b. Unusual reactions to foods, drugs, animals, plants, or household products

Note sensitivity to egg albumin and reactions to certain immunizations.

  6. Current medications

    a. Name, dose, schedule, duration, and reason for administration

Assess parents' knowledge of correct dosage of common drugs, such as acetaminophen; note underusage or overusage.

  7. Immunizations

    a. Name, number of doses, ages when given

    b. Occurrence of reaction

    c. Administration of horse or other foreign serum, gamma globulin, or blood transfusion

May refer to immunizations as "baby shots."

Whenever possible, confirm information by checking medical or school records.

  8. Growth and development

    a. Weight at birth, 6 months, 1 year, and present

    b. Dentition

      (1) Age of eruption/shedding

      (2) Number

      (3) Problems with teething

    c. Age of head control, sitting unsupported, walking, first words

    d. Present grade in school, scholastic achievement

    e. Interaction with peers and adults

    f. Participation in organized activities, such as scouts, sports, and so on

Compare parents' responses with own observations of child's achievement and results from objective tests, such as DDST or DASE

School and social history can be more thoroughly explored under Family Assessment.

9. Habits
  a. Behavior patterns
    (1) Nail biting
    (2) Thumb sucking
    (3) Pica
    (4) Rituals, such as "security blanket"
    (5) Unusual movements (headbanging, rocking)
    (6) Temper tantrums

Assess parents' attitudes toward habits and any remedies used to curtail them, such as punishment for bed-wetting.

  b. Activities of daily living
    (1) Hour of sleep and arising
    (2) Duration of nocturnal sleep/naps
    (3) Age of toilet training
    (4) Pattern of stools and urination; occurrence of enuresis

Record child's usual terms for defecation and urination.

    (5) Type of exercise
  c. Use/abuse of drugs, alcohol, coffee, or cigarettes

With adolescents, estimate the quantity of drugs used.

  d. Usual disposition; response to frustration

Review of Systems (ROS)

To elicit information concerning any potential health problem.

1. **General**—overall state of health, fatigue, recent or unexplained weight gain or loss, period of time for either, contributing factors (change of diet, illness, altered appetite), exercise tolerance, fevers

(time of day), chills, night sweats (unrelated to climatic conditions), frequent infections, general ability to carry out activities of daily living

Explain relevance of questioning to parents (similar to pregnancy section) in comprising total health history of child.

Make positive statements about each system, for example, "Mother denies headaches, bumping into objects, squinting, or excessive rubbing of eyes." Use terms parents are likely to understand, such as "bruises" for ecchymoses.

2. **Integument**—pruritus, pigment or other color changes, acne, eruptions, rashes (location), tendency to bruising, petechiae, excessive dryness, general texture, disorders or deformities of nails, hair growth or loss, hair color change (for adolescent, use of hair dyes or other potentially toxic substances, such as hair straighteners)

3. **Head**—headaches, dizziness, injury (specific details)

4. **Eyes**—visual problems (ask about behaviors that indicate blurred vision, such as bumping into objects, clumsiness, sitting very close to television, holding a book close to the face, writing with head near desk, squinting, rubbing the eyes, bending the head in an awkward position), "cross-eye" (strabismus), eye infections, edema of lids, excessive tearing, use of glasses or contact lenses, date of last optic examination

5. **Nose**—nosebleeds (epistaxis), constant or frequent running or stuffy nose, nasal obstruction (difficulty in breathing), sense of smell

6. **Ears**—earaches, discharge, evidence of hearing loss (ask about behaviors such as need to repeat requests, loud speech, inattentive behavior), results of any previous auditory testing

7. **Mouth**—mouth breathing, gum bleeding, toothaches, toothbrushing, use of fluoride, difficulty with teething (symptoms), last visit to dentist (especially if temporary dentition is complete), response to dentist

8. **Throat**—sore throats, difficulty in swallowing, choking (especially when chewing food, which may be caused by poor chewing habits), hoarseness or other voice irregularities
9. **Neck**—pain, limitation of movement, stiffness, difficulty in holding head straight (torticollis), thyroid enlargement, enlarged nodes or other masses
10. **Chest**—breast enlargement, discharge, masses, enlarged axillary nodes (for adolescent female, ask about breast self-examination)
11. **Respiratory**—chronic cough, frequent colds (number per year), wheezing, shortness of breath at rest or on exertion, difficulty in breathing, sputum production, infections (pneumonia, tuberculosis), date of last chest x-ray examination; date of last tuberculin test and type of reaction, if any
12. **Cardiovascular**—cyanosis or fatigue on exertion, history of heart murmur or rheumatic fever, anemia, date of last blood count, blood type, recent transfusion
13. **Gastrointestinal**—(much of this in regard to appetite, food tolerance, and elimination habits has been asked elsewhere) concentrate on nausea, vomiting (if not associated with eating, it may indicate brain tumor or increased intracranial pressure), jaundice or yellowing skin or sclera, belching, flatulence, recent change in bowel habits (blood in stools, change of color, diarrhea, or constipation)
14. **Genitourinary**—pain on urination, frequency, hesitancy, urgency, hematuria, nocturia, polyuria, unpleasant odor of urine, direction and force of stream, discharge, change in size of scrotum, date of last urinalysis (for adolescent, sexually transmitted disease, type of treatment; for adolescent male, ask about testicular self-examination)

15. **Gynecologic**—menarche, date of last menstrual period, regularity or problems with menstruation, vaginal discharge, pruritus, date and result of last Pap test (include obstetric history as discussed under Birth History when applicable), if sexually active, type of contraception
16. **Musculoskeletal**—weakness, clumsiness, lack of coordination, unusual movements, back or joint stiffness, muscle pains or cramps, abnormal gait, deformity, fractures, serious sprains, activity level
17. **Neurologic**—seizures, tremors, dizziness, loss of memory, general affect, fears, nightmares, speech problems, any unusual habits
18. **Endocrine**—intolerance to weather changes, excessive thirst, excessive sweating, salty taste to skin, signs of early puberty

Nutrition History

To elicit information about adequacy of child's dietary intake and eating patterns.

Family Medical History

To identify the presence of genetic traits or diseases that have familial tendencies; to assess family habits and exposure to a communicable disease that may affect family members.

Choose terms wisely when asking about child's parentage; for example, inquire about paternal history by referring to the child's "father" rather than mother's husband; use term "partner" rather than spouse.

1. Family pedigree and guidelines for construction

A pedigree is a pictorial representation or diagram of a family tree to visualize patterns of disease transmission

2. Familial diseases and congenital anomalies, such as heart disease, hypertension, cancer, diabetes mellitus, obesity, congenital anomalies, allergy, asthma, tuberculosis, sickle cell disease, mental retardation, convulsions, insanity or other emotional problems, syphilis, or rheumatic fever; indicate symptoms, treatment, and sequelae
3. Family habits, such as smoking or chemical use
4. Geographic location, such as recent travel or contact with foreign visitors

Important for identification of endemic diseases.

Family Personal/Social History

To gain an understanding of the family's structure and function.

Sexual History

To elicit information concerning young person's concerns or activities and any pertinent data regarding adults' sexual activity that influences child.

1. Sexual concerns/activity of youngster
2. Sexual concerns/activity of adults if warranted

Sexual history is an essential component of preadolescents' and adolescents' health assessment.

Degree of investigation into parents' sexual history depends on its relevance to the child's health. It may be limited to family planning concerns or it may be more detailed if overt sexual activity or abuse is suspected.

Investigate toward end of history when rapport is greatest.

Respect sensitive and complex nature of questioning.

 Give parents and youngster option of discussing sexual matters alone with nurse.

 Assure confidentiality.

 Clarify terms such as "sexually active" or "having sex."

 Refer to sexual contacts as "partners," not "girlfriends" or "boyfriends," to avoid biasing discussion of homosexual activity.

Discussion may flow easily after review of genitourinary tract, such as asking female about menstruation or male about urinary problems.

Suggestions for beginning discussion include:

 "Tell me about your social life."

 "Who are your closest friends?"

 "Is there one very special friend?"

 "Some teenagers have decided to have sex. What do you think about that?"

 Take detailed history of all contacts if sexually transmitted disease is suspected or diagnosed.

Patient Profile (P/P)

To summarize the interviewer's overall impression of the child's and family physical, psychologic, and socioeconomic background.

1. Health status
2. Psychologic status
3. Socioeconomic status

A comprehensive summary often identifies nursing diagnoses based on subjective and objective findings.

ADULT ASSESSMENT
ADULT HEALTH HISTORY
Taking the History

The following outline of what to include when taking a client history should be viewed not as a rigid structure but a general guideline. Since you are beginning your relationship with the client at this point, pay attention to this relationship, as well as to the information you seek in the history. Be friendly and show respect for the client. Choose a comfortable setting, and help the client get settled. Maintain eye contact, and use a conversational tone. Begin by introducing yourself and explaining your role. Help the client understand why you are taking the history and how it will be used. Once the history proceeds, explore positive responses with additional questions: where, when, what, how, and why. Be sensitive to the client's emotions at all times.

Chief Complaint

The problem or symptom: reason for visit

Duration of problem

Client information: age, gender, marital status, previous hospital admissions, occupation

Other complaints: secondary issues, fears, concerns, what made the client seek care

From Seidel HM and others: *Mosby's physical examination handbook,* St Louis, 1995, Mosby.

Present Problem

Chronologic ordering: sequence of events client has experienced

State of health just before the onset of the present problem

Complete description of the first symptom: time and date of onset, location, movement

Possible exposure to infection or toxic agents

If symptoms intermittent, describe typical attack: onset, duration, symptoms, variations, inciting factors, exacerbating factors, relieving factors

Impact of illness on lifestyle, on ability to function; limitations imposed by illness

"Stability" of the problem: intensity variations, improvement, worsening, staying the same

Immediate reason for seeking attention, particularly for long-standing problem

Review of appropriate system when there is a conspicuous disturbance of a particular organ or system

Medications: current and recent, dosage of prescriptions, home remedies, nonprescription medications

Review of chronology of events for each problem: client's confirmations and corrections

Past Medical History

General health and strength

Childhood illnesses: measles, mumps, whooping cough, chickenpox, smallpox, scarlet fever, acute rheumatic fever, diphtheria, poliomyelitis

Major adult illnesses: tuberculosis, hepatitis, diabetes, hypertension, myocardial infarction, tropical or parasitic diseases, other infections, any nonsurgical hospital admissions

Immunizations: poliomyelitis, diphtheria, pertussis, and tetanus toxoid, influenza, cholera, typhus, typhoid, bacille Calmette-Guérin (BCG), HBV, last PPD or other skin tests; unusual reactions to immunizations; tetanus or other antitoxin made with horse serum

Surgery: dates, hospital, diagnosis, complications

Serious injuries: resulting disability (document fully for injuries with possible legal implications)

Limitation of ability to function as desired as a result of past events

Medications: past, current and recent medications; dosage of prescription; home remedies and nonprescription medications

Allergies: especially to medications, but also to environmental allergens and foods

Transfusions: reactions, date, and number of units transfused

Emotional status: mood disorders, psychiatric treatment

Children: birth, developmental milestones, childhood diseases, immunizations

Family History

Relatives with similar illness

Immediate family: ethnicity, health, cause of and age at death

History of disease: heart disease, high blood pressure, hypercholesterolemia, cancer, tuberculosis, stroke, epilepsy, diabetes, gout, kidney disease, thyroid disease, asthma and other allergic states; forms of arthritis; blood diseases; sexually transmitted diseases; other familial diseases

Spouse and children: age, health

Hereditary disease: history of grandparents, aunts, uncles, siblings, cousins; consanguinity

Personal and Social History

Personal status: birthplace, where raised; home environment: parental divorce or separation, socioeconomic class, cultural background; education; position in family; marital status; general life satisfaction; hobbies and interests; sources of stress and strain

Habits: nutrition and diet, regularity and patterns of eating and sleeping; exercise: quantity and type; quantity of coffee, tea, tobacco; alcohol; illicit drugs: frequency, type, amount; breast or testicular self-examination

Sexual history: concerns with sexual feelings and performance; frequency of intercourse, ability to achieve orgasm, number and variety of partners

Home conditions: housing, economic condition, type of health insurance if any; pets and their health

Occupation: description of usual work and present work if different; list of job changes; work conditions and hours; physical and mental strain; duration of employment; present and past exposure to heat and cold, industrial toxins, especially lead, arsenic, chromium, asbestos, beryllium, poisonous gases, benzene, and polyvinyl chloride or other carcinogens and teratogens; any protective devices required, for example, goggles or masks

Environment: travel and other exposure to contagious diseases, residence in tropics, water and milk supply, other sources of infection if applicable

Military record: dates and geographic area of assignments

Religious preference: determine any religious proscriptions concerning medical care

Cost of care: resources available to patient, financial worries, candid discussion of issues

Review of Systems

General constitutional symptoms: fever, chills, malaise, fatigability, night sweats; weight (average, preferred, present, change)

Diet: appetite, likes and dislikes, restrictions (because of religion, allergy, or disease), vitamins and other supplements, use of caffeine-containing beverages (coffee, tea, cola); an hour-by-hour detailing of food and liquid intake—sometimes a written diary covering several days of intake may be necessary

Skin, hair, and nails: rash or eruption, itching, pigmentation or texture change; excessive sweating, abnormal nail or hair growth; in children, eczema or seborrhea

Musculoskeletal: joint stiffness, pain, restriction of motion, swelling, redness, heat, bony deformity

Head and neck:

General: frequent or unusual headaches, their location, dizziness, syncope, severe head injuries; periods of loss of consciousness (momentary or prolonged)

Eyes: visual acuity, blurring, diplopia, photophobia, pain, recent change in appearance or vision; glaucoma, use of eye drops or other eye medications; history of trauma or familial eye disease

Ears: hearing loss, pain, discharge, tinnitus, vertigo; in children, otitis media

Nose: sense of smell, frequency of colds, obstruction, epistaxis, postnasal discharge, sinus pain; in children, mouth breathing

Throat and mouth: hoarseness or change in voice; frequent sore throats, bleeding or swelling of gums; recent tooth abscesses or extractions; soreness of tongue or buccal mucosa ulcers; disturbance of taste

Endocrine: thyroid enlargement or tenderness, heat or cold intolerance, unexplained weight change, diabetes, polydipsia, polyuria, changes in facial or body hair, increased hat and glove size, skin striae

Males: puberty onset, erections, emissions, testicular pain, libido, infertility

Females:

Menses: onset, regularity, duration and amount of flow, dysmenorrhea, last period, intermenstrual discharge or bleeding, itching, date of last Pap smear, age at menopause, libido, frequency of intercourse, sexual difficulties, infertility

Pregnancies: number, miscarriages, abortions, duration of pregnancy, each type of delivery, any complications during any pregnancy or postpartum period or with neonate; use of oral or other contraceptives

Breasts: pain, tenderness, discharge, lumps, galactorrhea, mammograms (screening or diagnostic), frequency of breast self-examination

Chest and lungs: pain related to respiration, dyspnea, cyanosis, wheezing, cough, sputum (character and quantity), hemoptysis, night sweats, exposure to TB; date and result of last chest x-ray examination

Heart and blood vessels: chest pain or distress, precipitating causes, timing and duration, character; relieving factors; palpitations, dyspnea, orthopnea (number of pillows needed), edema, claudication, hypertension, previous myocardial infarction, estimate of exercise tolerance, past ECG or other cardiac tests

Hematologic: anemia, tendency to bruise or bleed easily, thromboses, thrombophlebitis, any known abnormality of blood cells, transfusions

Lymph nodes: enlargement, tenderness, suppuration

Gastrointestinal: appetite, digestion, intolerance for any class of foods, dysphagia, heartburn, nausea, vomiting, hematemesis, regularity of bowels, constipation, diarrhea, change in stool color or contents (clay-colored, tarry, fresh blood, mucus, undigested food), flatulence, hemorrhoids, hepatitis, jaundice, dark urine; history of ulcer, gallstones, polyps, tumor; previous x-ray examinations (where, when, findings)

Genitourinary: dysuria, flank or suprapubic pain, urgency, frequency, nocturia, hematuria, polyuria, hesitancy, dribbling, loss in force of stream, passage of stone; edema of face, stress incontinence, hernias, sexually transmitted disease (inquire type and symptoms, and results of serologic test for syphilis, if known)

Neurologic: syncope, seizures, weakness or paralysis, abnormalities of sensation or coordination, tremors, loss of memory

Psychiatric: depression, mood changes, difficulty concentrating, nervousness, tension, suicidal thoughts, irritability, sleep disturbances

ELDERLY ASSESSMENT
IMPORTANT ASPECTS OF HEALTH HISTORY IN THE ELDERLY
Social History
Living arrangements

Relationships with family and friends

Economic status

Abilities to perform activities of daily living

Social activities and hobbies

Mode of transportation

Past Medical History
Previous surgical procedures

Major illnesses and hospitalizations

Immunization status

    Influenza, pneumococcal, tetanus

Tuberculosis history and testing

Medications (use the "brown bag" technique; see text)

    Previous allergies

    Knowledge of current medication regimen

    Compliance

Perceived beneficial or adverse drug effects

Systems Review
Ask questions about general symptoms that may indicate treatable underlying disease such as fatigue, anorexia, weight loss, and insomnia

Attempt to elicit key symptoms in each organ system, including:

From Kane R, Ouslander J, Abrass I: *Essentials of clinical geriatrics,* ed 3, New York, 1994, McGraw-Hill.

System	Key symptoms
Respiratory	Increasing dyspnea
	Persistent cough
Cardiovascular	Orthopnea
	Edema
	Angina
	Claudication
	Palpitations
	Dizziness
	Syncope
Gastrointestinal	Difficulty chewing
	Dysphagia
	Abdominal pain
	Change in bowel habit
Genitourinary	Frequency
	Urgency
	Nocturia
	Hesitancy, intermittent stream, straining to void
	Incontinence
	Hematuria
	Vaginal bleeding
Musculoskeletal	Focal or diffuse pain
	Focal or diffuse weakness
Neurological	Visual disturbances (transient or progressive)
	Progressive hearing loss
	Unsteadiness and/or falls
	Transient focal symptoms
Psychological	Depression
	Anxiety and/or agitation
	Paranoia
	Forgetfulness and/or confusion

SITUATIONAL ASSESSMENT
ACTIVITIES OF DAILY LIVING ASSESSMENT

I. Introduction
   - A. Definition: Activities of daily living are those that a person performs on his own behalf in maintaining life, health, and well-being
   - B. Nursing assessment of client needs and functional abilities
     1. Determine ability to communicate verbally and non-verbally
     2. Assess desire to engage in self-assessment and self-care
     3. Medical history relevant to disability and preexisting health status
     4. Social history
     5. Home responsibilities
     6. Home accessibility
     7. Education
     8. Vocational status
     9. Avocational testing
     10. Transportation issues
     11. Endurance and level of fatigue

II. Evaluation of activities of daily living
   - A. Assess client's status using predetermined indicators and project discharge goals with evaluation of ADL
     1. Use of assistive devices
     2. Ability to secure own equipment
     3. Toileting/cleansing
     4. Bathing (washing and drying)

From Mumma CAM, editor: *Rehabilitation nursing concepts and practice: a core curriculum,* ed 2, Skokie, Ill, 1987, Rehabilitation Nursing Foundation.

5. Care of teeth (brushing; denture care, including oral placement/removal and storage)
6. Hair care (shampooing, brushing, and combing)
7. Skin care
8. Grooming (social/psychological additions to general appearance/self-image enhancement)
9. Dressing/undressing, upper and lower extremities
10. Eating (preparing meals and feeding self)
11. Personal care clean-up activities
12. Social/psychological activities
13. Kitchen tasks
14. Homemaking tasks
15. Child care
16. Community skills
17. Communication skills
18. Recreational activities
19. Sexual activity/function

B. Review findings of other team members

III. Designed program to increase self-care abilities

A. Program should include:
1. Evaluation of client's current functional status, actual and potential problems
2. Precautions to be exercised in view of medical status
3. Client and family interactions and determination of primary caregiver
4. Discharge plans and particular needs of client
5. Treatment plan established with physicians, therapist, client, family, nurse, and other team members

B. Evaluate factors contributing to inability to perform activities of daily living

1. Situational or environmental factors (inaccessibility, sensory overload, etc.)
2. Complexity of task and sequencing
3. Impaired ability to focus attention on task
4. Primary or secondary illnesses, disabilities, or deficits
5. Visual neglect
6. Impaired balance
7. Impaired endurance; low activity tolerance due to fatigue
8. Sensation deficit
9. Coordination deficit
10. Perceptual deficit
11. Impaired judgment
12. Impaired memory
13. Communication deficit
14. Apraxia
15. Spasticity
16. Contracture
17. Pain
18. Paralysis
19. Paresis
20. Lack of one or more extremity(ies)
21. Visual impairment
22. Auditory impairment
23. Mobility deficit
24. Learning impairments
25. Psychological impairment
    a. Loss, grief, or depression
    b. Self-image deficit
    c. Motivation (role in self-initiation of care tasks)

C. Specific elements to consider in activities of daily living training
  1. Feeding
     a. Utensil, cup, plate management, and napkin use
     b. Tidiness/organization
     c. Awareness of swallowing, chewing, or pocketing problems
     d. Ability to handle different food consistencies, e.g., finger foods versus soups
     e. Mouth care after eating
  2. Bathing
     a. Assembling of items and appropriate equipment
     b. Management of caps, lids, sprays, etc.
     c. Facial cleansers and cosmetic application
     d. Shaving foam or soap application versus electric razor
     e. Shaving face, underarms, and/or legs
     f. Hair care
     g. Deodorant application
     h. Tooth/denture care
     i. Nail care
     j. Replacement of care items
     k. Location of bath facilities in hospital and home
     l. Transfer ability to bathtub or shower
  3. Dressing
     a. Selection of clothing
     b. Assembling of clothing
     c. Application of underwear
     d. Management of fasteners
     e. Application of trousers/slacks, belt or suspenders
     f. Management of buckles and zippers

    g. Application of pullover tops
    h. Application of shirt, jacket, dress (front opening), or tie
    i. Management of buttons
    j. Application of socks or stockings
    k. Application of shoes and tying laces
    l. Location of dressing activities; bed, sitting or standing
    m. Ability to care for and apply glasses, contact lenses, or hearing aid

4. Toileting and elimination management
    a. Transfer ability
    b. Clothing management
    c. Cognitive function
    d. Bowel and bladder control
    e. External devices: assembly, application, removal, and care of equipment
    f. Suppository insertion (include preparation of suppository and cleaning of insertion device if used)
    g. Post-toileting hygiene
    h. Timing of bowel program (morning or evening)
    i. Employment/school/home/environmental considerations
    j. Colostomy or ileal conduit care
    k. Performance of bladder management programs
    l. Accident management

ASSESSMENT DATA FOR PERSONS EXPERIENCING A LOSS

Name _____

Date _____

Age _____

1. Nature of the lost object (or person)
2. Meaning the lost object (or person) had for the mourner
3. Mourner's typical coping patterns
4. Mourner's social and cultural milieu
5. Mourner's attitude toward death (if applicable)
6. Special resources (support systems) the mourner possesses for coping with the loss
7. Factors that influence the mourning process:

    Importance of the lost object (or person) as a source of support

    Degree of ambivalence toward the lost object (or person)

    Age of the deceased (if applicable)

    Quantity and quality of other relationships

    Degree of preparation for the loss, which was

    Sudden _____

    Gradual _____

    Mourner's physical health

    Mourner's psychologic health

From Detherage KS, Johnson SS: Stress reduction and crisis intervention. In Edelman CL, Mandle CL, editors: *Health promotion throughout the lifespan,* ed 3, St Louis, 1994, Mosby.

CHILDBEARING ASSESSMENT
PRENATAL ASSESSMENT GUIDE
Aspects of Adaptation

Age

Initial response to pregnancy

Planned or unplanned pregnancy

Feelings about pregnancy

Desired family size

Perception of pregnancy affecting present activities and responsibilities

Perception of parenthood affecting future activities and plans

Current developmental task of pregnancy: coping mechanisms, fantasies about pregnancy, changes in mood and effect on others

Sexual functioning during pregnancy: changes, feelings, problems

Nature of verbal interest expressed about self and fetus

Preparations for prenatal classes (type, when completed), place of delivery, other children in mother's absence, and new sibling

Menstrual history: problems, last normal menstrual period, expected date of confinement

Height and prepregnancy weight

Past obstetric history: dates, course, outcomes

Present obstetric status: course, abdominal assessment, quickening, fetal heart sound, blood pressure, urinalysis, weight and pattern of gain, signs of any major complications of pregnancy

Past medical history: illness, date, treatment, outcome, surgery, childhood diseases, current immunization status, allergies, venereal disease, emotional problems

---

Modified from Becker C: *Obstet Gynecol Neonat Nurs,* Nov/Dec 1982 in Hancock LA et al: The prenatal period. In Edelman CL, Mandle CL, editors: *Health promotion throughout the lifespan,* ed 3, St Louis, 1994, Mosby.

Family medical history: illnesses, emotional problems, genetic defects
(both sides of family)

Loss of significant other in past year

Food intolerances (lactose, nausea and vomiting), food cravings, and
pica

Iron-vitamin-mineral dietary supplements used

Elimination patterns: changes, problems with remedies used

Pattern of rest, sleep: difficulties, remedies used

Aspects of Personal Belief System and Lifestyle

Date first sought prenatal care this pregnancy and in prior pregnancies

Reasons for seeking and receiving prenatal care

Beliefs about pregnancy and childbirth; cultural beliefs about child-
bearing (antepartum, intrapartum, postpartum)

Racial, ethnic group

Beliefs about role of father during pregnancy and labor and in child care

Perception of needs of fetus

Perception of needs of infant and proposed methods to meet these needs

Contraceptive history: methods used, failures or problems, knowledge
of alternate methods, willingness to use

Patterns of use of tobacco, alcohol, prescription and nonprescription
drugs, illegal drugs; perception of effects on health of self and fetus

Patterns of nutrient intake: food dislikes, history and method of dieting

Planned method of infant feeding; why chosen

Occupation: present, former, how long, work requirements, hazards,
amenities, plans regarding current occupation

Recreational activities: plans to continue, use of seat belt in car, pets
in home

Community activities

Perception of and prior experiences with health care personnel and
agencies

Date of last physical examination, including breast examination, Pap
smear, chest x-ray films, dental checkup

Breast self-examination done regularly; if not, interested in learning
about?

Aspects of Support

Address: how long there, housing accommodations, phone, plans to
move (when, where, why?)

Level of education and future plans regarding

Religious preference; normal or active involvement

Marital status; years married

Father of baby; age, occupation, educational level, racial and ethnic
group, religious preference

Family composition: household members

Communication patterns with significant others

Communication patterns with health personnel

Perception of support system (mate, family, friends, community agencies) available and willingness to use

Perception of meaning of this pregnancy to significant others; mate's
response to news of pregnancy

Type of prenatal service receiving and perception of its adequacy

Available transportation

Social service and community agencies involved with: how long and
contact person

Self-concept and perceived ability to cope with life situations

Body-image concept: prepregnant and current; response to physiologic
changes of pregnancy

Mate's response to body changes in pregnancy

Feelings about parenting woman received as a child; history of separation from mother

Prior experiences with infants; knowledge of infant care

Feelings about previous pregnancies, labor, puerperium, and mothering skills

Knowledge of reproduction, labor and delivery, and puerperium

OBSERVATIONS TO BE MADE AT POSTPARTUM CHECKUPS AND PEDIATRIC CHECKUPS

1. Does the mother have fun with the baby?
2. Does the mother establish eye contact (direct in face position) with the baby?
3. How does the mother talk to her baby? Is everything she expresses a demand?
4. Are most of her verbalizations about the child negative?
5. Does she remain disappointed over the child's sex?
6. What is the child's name? Where did it come from? When did they name the child?
7. Are the mother's expectations for the child's development far beyond the child's capabilities?
8. Is the mother very bothered by the baby's crying? How does she feel about the crying?
9. Does the mother see the baby as too demanding during feedings? Is she repulsed by the messiness? Does she ignore the baby's demands to be fed?
10. What is the mother's reaction to the task of changing diapers?
11. When the baby cries, does she or can she comfort him?
12. What was/is the husband's and/or family's reaction to the baby?
13. What kind of support is the mother receiving?
14. Are there sibling rivalry problems?
15. Is the husband jealous of the baby's drain on the mother's time and affection?
16. When the mother brings the child for checkups, does she get involved and take control over the baby's needs and what's going to

Modified from Kempe CH: Approaches to preventing child abuse, *Am J Dis Child* 130, 1976.

happen (during the examination and while in the waiting room) or does she relinquish control to the physician or nurse (undressing the child, holding him, allowing him to express his fears, etc.)?

17. Can attention be focused on the child in the mother's presence? Can the mother see something positive for her in that?

18. Does the mother make nonexistent complaints about the baby? Does she describe to you a child that you don't see there at all? Does she call with strange stories that the child has, for example, stopped breathing, turned color, or is doing something "on purpose" to aggravate the parent?

19. Does the mother make emergency calls for very small things, not major things?

PART II

TIPS FOR THE HOME VISIT

SAFETY GUIDELINES

1. Do not take your purse with you on visits. Lock it in your desk or file cabinet before leaving the office.
2. Keep the interior of the car free of personal belongings. If you must keep personal items in your car, lock them in the trunk before leaving the office parking lot.
3. Alert the family (when possible) that you are coming, and have them watch for you.
4. Have accurate directions to the street, building, apartment.
5. If the area is unfamiliar to you, check with your supervisor for more detailed information.
6. If you are driving alone, drive with the windows closed and all car doors locked.
7. As you approach your destination, carefully observe your surroundings, e.g., note location and activity of people; types and locations of cars; condition of buildings (abandoned or heavily congested buildings).
8. Park in a well-lighted and heavily traveled area.

Courtesy Visiting Nurse and Home Care, Inc, Waterbury, Conn.

9. Before getting out of the car, once again thoroughly check the surroundings. If you feel uneasy, do not get out of the car. Return to the office or call from a safe location.

10. Be alert at all times, from the moment you leave the office until you return.

PHASES AND ACTIVITIES OF A HOME VISIT

Phase	Activity
I. Initiation phase	Clarify source of referral for visit Clarify purpose for home visit Share information on reason and purpose of home visit with family
II. Previsit phase	Initiate contact with family Establish shared perception of purpose with family Determine family's willingness for home visit Schedule home visit Review referral and/or family record
III. In-home phase	Introduction of self and professional identity Social interaction to establish rapport Establish nurse-client relationship Implement nursing process
IV. Termination phase	Review visit with family Plan for future visits
V. Postvisit phase	Record visit Plan for next visit

Developed by C Loveland-Cherry; from Stanhope M, Lancastor J: *Community health nursing,* ed 4, St Louis, 1996, Mosby.

ESSENTIAL SUPPLIES AND EQUIPMENT
Home Visit Bag

1. Sphygmomanometer   ___
2. Stethoscope   ___
3. Thermometer   ___
   a. Oral   ___
   b. Rectal   ___
4. Scissors   ___
5. Forceps   ___
6. Epinephrine   ___
7. TB syringe/needle   ___
8. Soap   ___
9. Towels   ___
10. Apron   ___
11. Antiseptic wipes   ___
12. Tape measure   ___
13. Penlight   ___
14. Otoscope/ophthalmoscope (optional)   ___
15. Gloves/mask/eyeshield   ___

Additional Supplies/Equipment for Home Visit

1. Wound care supplies ——
   a. 4 × 4 ——
   b. 2 × 2 ——
   c. Kling ——
   d. Antiseptic solution ——
   e. Irrigation solution ——
   f. Other _____ ——
2. Asepto syringe ——
3. Intravenous therapy set-up ——
4. Catheter equipment ——
5. Suction catheter ——
6. Irrigation set-up ——
7. Enema ——
8. Ace bandages ——
9. Slings ——
10. Splints ——
11. CPR mask ——
12. Other _____ ——

From Stanhope M, Knollmueller R: *Handbook of community and home health nursing: tools for assessment, intervention, and education,* ed 2, St Louis, 1996, Mosby.

BAG TECHNIQUE

Follow agency policy and procedure for appropriate bag technique.

Review plan of care and/or physician's orders.

Check your bag for essential supplies and equipment to conduct home visit.

To prevent nurse-to-client, client-to-nurse, or client-to-client contamination, place bag on paper towels or newspaper.

Explain your actions to the client.

Wash hands before removing contents of bag.

Use good handwashing technique, and turn off faucets with paper towels.

Prepare a clean field with paper towels to lay out your equipment/supplies.

Follow universal precaution guidelines when providing home care.

Discard used supplies, syringes, and needles according to agency policy.

AFTER care is given, wash hands and clean equipment before repacking the bag.

Organize the bag for efficient use.

From Stanhope M, Knollmueller R: *Handbook of community and home health nursing: tools for assessment, intervention, and education,* ed 2, St Louis, 1996, Mosby.

HAND WASHING TECHNIQUE

1. Use a sink with warm running water, soap, and paper towels.
2. Push wristwatch and long uniform sleeves up above wrists. Remove jewelry, except a plain band, from fingers and arms.
3. Keep fingernails short and filed.
4. Inspect the surface of the hands and fingers for breaks or cuts in the skin and cuticles. Report such lesions when caring for highly susceptible clients.
5. Stand in front of the sink, keeping hands and uniform away from the sink surface. (If hands touch the sink during hand washing, repeat the process.) Use a sink where it is comfortable to reach the faucet.
6. Turn on the water. Turn on hand-operated faucets by covering the faucet with a paper towel.
7. Avoid splashing water against your uniform or clothes.
8. Regulate flow of water so the temperature is warm.
9. Wet hands and lower arms thoroughly under running water. Keep the hands and forearms lower than the elbows during washing.
10. Apply 1 ml of regular or 3 ml of antiseptic liquid soap to the hands, lathering thoroughly. If bar soap is used, hold it throughout the lathering period. Soap granules and leaflet preparations may be used.
11. Wash the hands, using plenty of lather and friction for at least 10 to 15 seconds. Interlace the fingers and rub the palms and back of hands with a circular motion at least 5 times each.
12. If areas underlying fingernails are soiled, clean them with fingernails of the other hand and additional soap or a clean orangewood stick. Do not tear or cut the skin under or around the nail.

Modified from Potter PA, Perry AG: *Fundamentals of nursing: concepts, process, and practice,* ed 3, St Louis, 1993, Mosby.

13. Rinse hands and wrists thoroughly, keeping hands down and elbows up.
14. Repeat steps 10 through 12 but extend the actual period of washing for 1-, 2-, and 3-minute hand washings.
15. Dry the hands thoroughly from the fingers up to the wrists and forearms.
16. Discard paper towel in proper receptacle.
17. To turn off a hand faucet, use a clean, dry paper towel.

Remember to treat the inside of your "black bag" as clean. Always wash hands before removing supplies and equipment from bag or putting clean supplies in the bag. Carry soap and paper towels in outside packets of your bag or at inner top.

TIPS ON DOCUMENTATION FOR HOME HEALTH
Basic Considerations

1. When appropriate, documentation should indicate client is homebound with specific notation of physical limitations or restrictions that would not allow leaving home. Notes should not indicate activities done outside the home except for physician or laboratory appointments. Some situations indicating homebound treatment follow:

   a. Fractures or disabilities that prevent ambulation without assistance or use of assistive aids, or that prevent weight bearing or the use of arms to open doors, etc.

   b. Shortness of breath with slight exertion as in chronic obstructive pulmonary disease (COPD) or chronic heart failure

   c. Weakness as result of surgery or illness or client being easily fatigued

   d. Dizziness, weakness, poor balance, or unsteady gait

   e. Incision, draining wound, or dressing changes

   f. Indwelling catheter

   g. Wheelchair or bed-bound

   h. Sensory deficiencies such as visual or auditory impairment or aphasia

   i. Paraplegia, quadriplegia, hemiplegia, numbness of extremities, paresis, or impaired peripheral circulation

   j. Mental confusion, extreme anxiety, or paranoia

   k. Obesity

   l. Severe pain

2. List all medical diagnoses on care plan because care may be needed for more than one condition; document the most acute diagnosis as the principal diagnosis, using onset date.
3. Indicate a date for each problem or nursing diagnosis in care plan.
4. Documentation should be succinct, descriptive, and relevant. Omit items or words that do not relate or contribute to the necessary information.
5. Omit words describing care given, such as:
   a. Use of chronic for acute exacerbation
   b. Use of monitor for assess or evaluate if condition has stabilized
   c. Use of reinforce instead of reinstruct for instruction
   d. Use of discussed instead of instructed
   e. Use of check instead of perform
   f. Use of observe instead of assess
   g. Use of words such as stabilized or reviewed instead of responding to treatment
6. Document what is wrong with client, not only client's progress or what is right with him or her. Indicate need for care, not that care is no longer needed, for example:
   Incorrect: respirations improving in rate, depth, and ease
   Correct: respirations remaining at 28 per minute with use of accessory muscles and presence of dyspnea
7. Document information in a factual, objective manner. Avoid injecting subjective information, for example:
   Incorrect: general weakness
   Correct: able to ambulate only 10 feet without fatigue and dizziness
   Incorrect: reddened area on right heel
   Correct: reddened area on right heel, measuring 1 cm in diameter

8. Document all care that relates to medical diagnoses and orders. Be specific and include all care and skills performed, for example: Instruct client to draw insulin into syringe, using sterile technique.

9. Document unstable states that require interventions such as medication or catheter changes, sterile irrigations, pulmonary physiotherapy, and others that need skilled nursing care. Make sure skilled care matches the diagnoses and physician orders.

10. Document exercise or other regimens that are performed to restore function lost because of condition being treated and described by medical diagnoses.

11. Document in the care plan the exact services being provided that require skilled, professional nursing care.

12. Indicate in the care plan the time frames in which care will be provided, such as two to three times per week or less, depending on condition and insurance parameters.

13. Document goal achievement with dates at least weekly on plan.

14. Each note should contain why the visit was needed; use specific information from assessment to affirm medical necessity and specific care given.

*Additional Considerations**

Do not document the following:

    Private sitter or companion

    Client trips

    Medications reviewed

    Repetitive teaching

    Lack of progress when progress should be seen; instead document
        inability to participate in therapy

Do document the following:

    Why client or family cannot be taught a procedure

    Poor comprehension of client or family

    Specific signs and symptoms of disease taught to client

    Therapeutic diet taught with sample menus

    Return demonstrations by client to evaluate level of competence

    Medications taught; teach one each visit

*Modified from Jaffe M, Skidmore-Roth L: *Home health nursing care plans,* St Louis, 1988, Mosby.